Homeopathic Remedies Beyond Avogadro's Number

An Observational Study of High Potency Homeopathic Particles

Acknowledgements

➢ Helios Homoeopathy Ltd at: 89 - 97 Camden Rd, Tunbridge Wells, Kent TN1 2QR [UK] for supplying all the remedies [except one- Medorrhinum 6x] that were used in the study

➢ JoAnn Jarvis, RN, DHM, for her consult, support and editing

➢ Janet Beegle Gay, for her support and editing

➢ Nansee Messenger, for her support and editing

➢ Rebecca Bieling, for her support and editing

➢ Robert Bieling, for his support and editing

➢ Richard Huemer, M.D., consultant

➢ James Brownlow, PhD, consultant, back cover

➢ Sue Liberto, for taking the photograph of the author and illustrator

Preface Note:

Since this research was first published in "The California Homeopath; Journal of the California Homeopathic Medical Society", I have wanted to clarify that I did a Scientific Observational Study as a research project.

I have decided to expand on some of the explanations and add in some new information. Part of this new information is the method I used to locate the homeopathic micrometer pieces, since I found it impossible to just zoom in and see them. I had to zoom in in stages. This is explained in more detail within this publication. I also added in the two remedies that were included in my original study, but were not in the first published work due to space.

Dr. Shirl Airov-Bieling

Table of Contents

v

Introduction

The original purpose of this study was to determine through a scientific observational study, if there was a vital substance in homeopathic remedies found in high potencies. The definition of Potency: It is the level strength or vitality of the homeopathic remedy, which would be determined by how that remedy was processed. A vital substance, in this case, is defined as a substance that that is alive and energetic in the remedies to help heal a person of a certain ailment. Since the remedies are diluted and processed many, many times when they are made into a high potency, the question has arose about there being any vital substance of the homeopathic remedy left in these higher potencies. Some in the scientific community say that when you dilute something beyond a certain point, a point which is called Avogadro's number, that there are no particles of substance left. [Avogadro's number is the number of particles in one mole of substance.] But the homeopathic remedies have worked and been shown to be vital well beyond this point. The reason[s] why homeopathic remedies are vital in these higher potencies is still in question. The Nanoparticle research has proven that there are particles of homeopathic substance beyond Avogadro's number[1]. It was yet to be shown that these particles are vital and to see pictures of homeopathic particles.

A study was read where there was a clustering of molecules in high dilutions of substances.[2] So a plan to try to observe this phenomenon, using a Phenom Scanning Electron Microscope [SEM], which is a 'desktop' model of an SEM, was devised, as seen below.

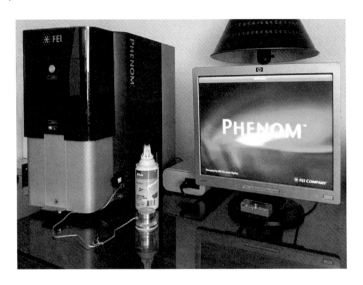

Phenom Scanning Electron Microscope©

While this SEM is still large [@200 lbs.], it was not strong enough to magnify to a molecular level. But since the SEM is a VERY expensive toy, it was decided to observe what could be found at the Phenom SEM's level of magnification, which is on a micrometer [μ] level.

I set up an observational study where the scans were taken, observed and/or analyzed. In the beginning, when the study was set up, I took the scans randomly since nothing was known about what would be found. As the study progressed, more became known about what to look for in the scans and which scan pictures to take. This was because I devised a way to find the interesting shapes without overheating the microscope and getting totally frustrated. I would first magnify the sample just a little; maybe up to 1000x magnification. If I saw something that looked like it had possibilities, I would up the magnification to 5,000x. Then, if there was still an interesting shape, I would up the magnification to 14,000x magnification. I found that if I just went straight to the 14,000x magnification, I most likely would not locate the tiniest interesting shapes, which were usually the ones I wanted to see. These interesting tiny certain shapes that were emerging with this method, did not look like just sugar, or just alcohol treated sugar as the base scan picture showed. This allowed the research to progress with more targeted scans captured, instead of just randomly taking scans of everything, and finding very little.

The scan photos of the remedy powders were analyzed after all of the remedies that were to be scanned were taken.

The scans showed the base sugar, impurities, dust, and some very interesting other structures that, though analysis, were concluded to be the homeopathic remedies combined with the alcohol/water base. This will be elaborated in detail within the body of these writings.

To my happy surprise, the results turned out to be very fascinating, since one could observe homeopathic substances even at the 1M potency level. Because of these observations, the study was continued to see if these observations could be found in other homeopathic remedies, and also to see if these homeopathic substances could be found in various higher potency remedies.

The Study

Chapter 1

The Study

The Phenom SEM was used to observe and record the findings, and impressions of a study of ten different homeopathic remedies. These were compared on four potency levels. The remedies used were applied to a sugar lactose powder by a pharmaceutical lab[3]. In Homeopathy, base diluents of water and alcohol are used to make the homeopathic remedies. These diluents are applied to sugar pellets. The pellets are made of a sugar substrate, but for this study, the sugar used was in a powdered form of lactose. A SEM cannot have samples that have any moisture in them. An environmental scanning electron microscope, ESEM, can have a little bit of moisture, but one could still not scan liquids. Liquids can be used for other studies, or experiments, such as the ones that have identified nanometer homeopathic particles. Even the larger, more powerful ESEMs could not use the liquid samples. This is why powdered samples were used.

The first scans of this study are of the plain basic product of alcohol/water applied to the lactose powder, and a plain unmedicated lactose sugar powder. These base scans are the beginning reference points. All the remedies, base and sugar were scanned at 14,000x magnification of a 17.2µm spot and captured into pictures. The ten remedies used were: Apis mellifica, Arnica Montana, Chamomilla, Gelsemium sempervirens, Lachesis mutus, Medorrhinum, Natrum muriaticum, Ruta graveolens, Sepia and Sulfur [Sulfur is the scientific spelling; this is also spelled sulphur in some homeopathic literature]. Each remedy was observed at a 6x, 30c, 200c, and 1M potency level. There were 15 to 20 scans captured for each potency level for each of the ten remedies. There were also approximately 15-20 scans done of the plain sugar lactose powder and the alcohol/water base on the sugar powder.

Most of the structures that were identified as pieces of homeopathic remedies were found in and among the pieces of sugar, and sometimes unidentified objects [which might have been impurities or dust]. Many of the times the pieces were located near larger structures, such as sugar. The first picture below is of the sample stub before the electron scanning by the microscope starts. It is a picture of 24x magnification, of the Apis 30c powder applied to the stub. The part that is circled in green is an example of an area where the remedy might have been found. The process I used to find these structures, which I outlined in the introduction, was as follows: I would first magnify the scan to about 5000x magnification, to see if any interesting pieces were located in that particular spot. If I found some pieces of interest, I would then up the magnification to about 10,000x with the located particles in the middle of the scan. If the site was still of interest at the 10,000x magnification, I would then position the pieces of interest into the center of the scan again. Then I would up the magnification up to the target of level 14,000x and see if the structures were what I had been searching for. If they were, I would make a copy of the scan.

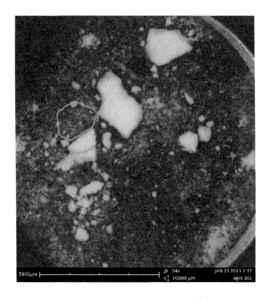

Apis 30 stub- 24x magnification scan©

The second picture is of the sample stub, the microscope's stub holder, black carbon sticky pads to hold the sample, [such as the remedy powders] tweezers to hold the stub, and a box to hold stubs.

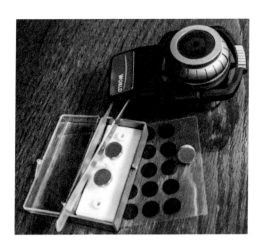

Picture of things used with the SEM©

Homeopathic pieces were not found in all the scans. Yet, in review of other studies, and taking into consideration the limits of this SEM used, more pieces of homeopathic chunks might have been present. Those pieces might be smaller; even on a nanometer scale. But they would not have been detected because of the limits of this study. The higher the potency of the homeopathic, the smaller, yet more defined the homeopathic structures seemed to become in a lot of the different remedies.

The sizes of each of the remedy pieces varied with from one remedy to another. Sulfur had the largest pieces, and Arnica montana seemed to be the next largest. There are also differences in shapes, hardness, and how much the remedy seemed to mix with the alcohol. Each remedy had one or two distinctive structures, except Sulfur, which had more than two.

The Theory of Why There is Vital Substance in All Levels of Potency in Homeopathic Remedies

Chapter 2

The Theory of How the High Potency Homeopathic Remedies Retain Their Vitality

The following theory of how high potency homeopathic remedies are still vital and active, was formulated from the observations that were made. But let us first give an explanation of how homeopathic remedies are produced.

All remedies are made from a mother substance by extracting, or triturating and then extracting the base homeopathic substance. This mother ingredient is processed by dilution with alcohol/water. The substance is then shaken with forcible impact. This shaking with impact or pounding process is called succussion. A 6x (ratio of 1:10) potency remedy will be diluted and then succussed 60 times, and a 20c (ratio of 1:100) potency remedy, 200 times and succussed, and so on for all the potency levels. At each new potency level, the previous potency is used and diluted again with the alcohol/water diluent. Once again this is succussed to reach the next highest potency. This very processed liquid remedy is then usually applied to the sugar substrate. The sugar lactose used in this study or sugar pellet is used as a carrier on which the liquid remedy is applied, and so is not part of the potentizing process. The following is a statement of the theory that has been reached in this study:

The substance of origin in the homeopathic remedies over 12c or 24x formulations are not lost due to dilution because

of the alcohol used and because of the succussion done between each new level of potency. The method used to create each new homeopathic potency level of diluting the liquid in an alcohol/water base, combined with the succussion used in a very controlled fashion, creates an extracted solution on each new potency level of the whole diluted homeopathic substance. Succussing creates a stronger extraction on each new potency level. This means there is a new homeopathic substance in the new, or next level of potency, because the processing of the dilution has created it.

Alcohol is used in scientific laboratories to create extractions because it is a universal solvent. Agitation is used as another extraction method in medical laboratories. The harder, faster pounding and shaking used in the extensive succussion method [a type of agitation] would cause the extraction process to occur faster and the extract to be stronger. Plus, the succussion would make the structures more defined. In other words, this second might process preserve the homeopathic, so it is found as an extraction in the next potency level's formula. Therefore, the homeopathic particles would be in a new solution for every new potency level. This might be the scientific reason why the remedies are not being diluted out of the liquid.

The two stage processing of substance would cause the homeopathic particles to be in a new solution for every new potency level. This might be the scientific reason why the remedies are not being diluted out of the liquid. The remedies are being changed into a new extracted solution, which contains homeopathic structures that are usually smaller, yet more defined, for each new potency level. The remedies are being changed into a new extracted solution, which contains homeopathic structures that are usually smaller, yet they seem more defined, for each new potency level.

The changes to the remedies by the extracting alcohol and succussion causes can be seen in the scans. A discussion of the observations that led to this theory is given here in detail. All of the remedies that were observed had similarities within the scans, which looked like the plain lactose and the alcohol/water base. These similar characteristics were in all the homeopathic remedies scans on all levels. But, most of the remedy scan also had individual qualities which probably contained the properties of the original substances, which was the substance that each of the remedies were made from. The visual qualities are sometimes strikingly different from the alcohol/water and the sugar base properties. An important point is that the different features that seem to be particular to the remedy's properties were found in the 6x remedies scans on up to the 1M remedies scans. In addition, many of the scans of the homeopathic substances appeared different from each other. In other words, the Arnica montana scans have observable differences from the Medorrhinum and other remedy scans that are not Arnica montana. Each remedy has distinct characteristics that distinguish it from the others.

The Analysis of the Scans

Base Scans:

Lactose Sugar Scans
&
Alcohol/Water Scans

Chapter 3

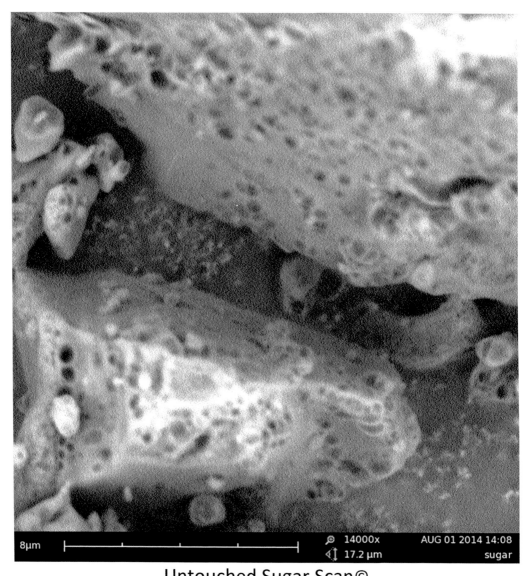

Untouched Sugar Scan©

Sugar

The first base scan is of the plain powdered sugar lactose, which is the inert material to which all the different remedy solutions are applied in this study by the pharmaceutical lab.

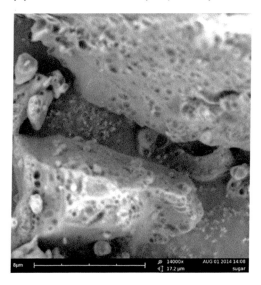

Sugar Lactose Powder Scan©

Many of the plain sugar lactose scans seem to have a texture that reminds one of the crevices found in pictures of moon craters. Some of the crevices are deep and some are shallow. These sugar formations are sometimes separate structures found in the scanned pictures, and sometimes they appear attached to other structures in the scan. The above scan shows both examples. There were groups of scans taken for each of the remedies in the study. Pockmarks can be found in all of the remedies scanned. But these pieces were not always in the scans that contained the remedy formations. Some remedies pieces did not have pockmarks. They were smooth. Some had remedy marks that were deeper and looked more eruptive than the sugar pockmarks. This suggests that some of the remedies might have their own particular type of pockmarks and some do not have any marks. Some of the sugar pieces had rough surfaces on their chunks, and others were smoother. But some of the remedies were smoother than all the sugar structures that had some smoothness. The lactose sugar structures were varied in size, but many of the pieces were large; larger than all the homeopathic remedy formations. Sugar pieces could be found all over the scan pictures. They were not necessarily the smaller structures tucked into the corners near the larger pieces, which is where most of the homeopathic remedy pieces were found. Note the background of the sample stub structure used in the microscope does show up as little bumps in all the scans due to how the sample was prepared. Plus there was probably some small amount of dust particles in all the scans. There were differences in the lactose sugar structures from the homeopathic remedies pieces that could be observed upon careful examination. Also note that all the homeopathic remedies, after their dilution and processing, are applied to the sugar. Thus, some of the sugar properties would probably be present in most, if not all, the scans of the remedies. Each remedy seemed to react to the sugar differently, according to its own traits. [Note: all the scan pictures are in the text except those marked "untouched" are 'cleaned up' in Photoshop. The cleaned-up changes are things like making the pictures despeckled, so the pictures would be clear enough to view. <u>No other enhancements were made</u>.]

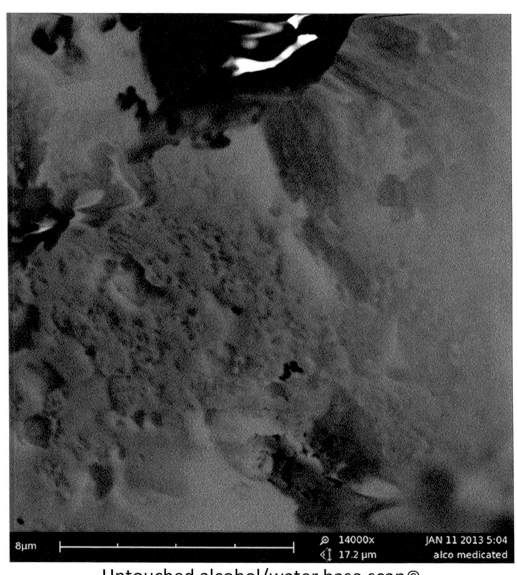

| 8μm | | ⌀ 14000x | JAN 11 2013 5:04 |
| | | ⬍↕ 17.2 μm | alco medicated |

Untouched alcohol/water base scan©

Alcohol/Water Base

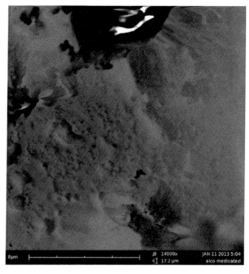

Alcohol/Water applied to the Sugar Lactose©

The plain alcohol/water base solution was added to the lactose sugar at the laboratories that made most of the homeopathic remedies used in this study[1]. These scans are called medicated scans, since they have alcohol added, but do not have any remedy added to them. The alcohol/water on the lactose sugar seems to alter most of the sugar crevices, which results in a smoother visual effect. This smoothness can be seen on all the scans of all the remedies. One particular aspect of this smoothed out sugar in the plain medicated scans is that there are few defined shapes. The scan looks as if all the parts are melted together. This melting together of the sugar into one large piece was only found in the medicated alcohol/water sugar base scans.

The Remedies

Apis mellifica 6x Remedy

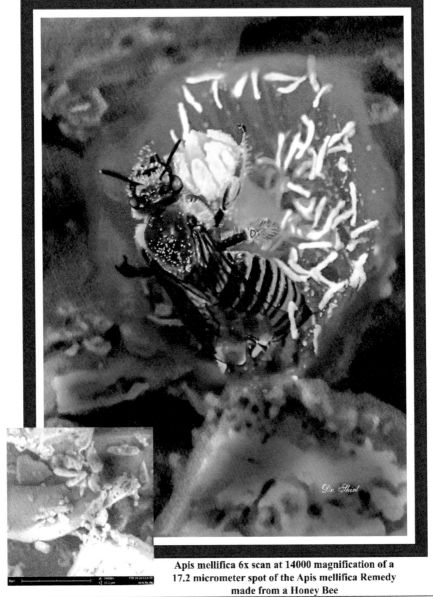

Apis mellifica 6x scan at 14000 magnification of a
17.2 micrometer spot of the Apis mellifica Remedy
made from a Honey Bee

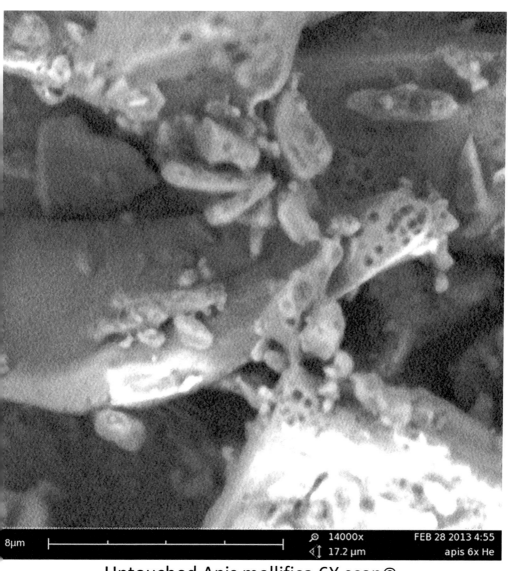

Untouched Apis mellifica 6X scan©

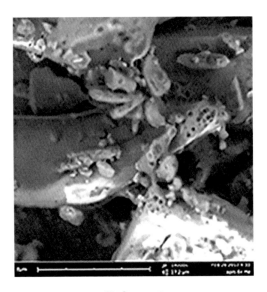

Apis mellifica 6x scan©

The Apis mellifica [commonly called Apis] scans show structures that have pieces that have areas that are smooth with distinct round edges. The alcohol scans have the smooth areas but not those same distinctive edges. Note the creviced areas in Apis 6x. These crevices are isolated and not found throughout the whole structure such as in a lot of the sugar scans. There are structures in many Apis scans that look similar to a blunted swollen tip. The 6x scan shown above has these structures outlined in green, to give clarity to the description. Pieces with rounded edges and a blunted swollen tip are present in all of the potency levels of the Apis scans: the 6x, 30c, 200c, and 1M. Some of the scans are more pointed than others, but the trait still seems to be present throughout the Apis remedy scans. These structures seemed to be particular to the Apis scans, and not the other remedy scans. Thus one might assume that they are characteristic of the Apis remedy. It seems there is a physiochemical liquid which is made of the combination of the Apis and the alcohol/water solution. [Physiochemical means there is a physical and chemical combination] The whole combination [Apis/alcohol/water] liquid is then added to the sugar lactose to form the remedy's formation. This means the structure seems to have the physical and chemical properties, or the physiochemical properties, of the alcohol/water and the Apis extract contained within the piece. Plain sugar like pieces show up in most of the scans in all the remedies, as seen in the bottom lower right and a small piece attached to the large Apis structure in the Apis mellifica 6x scan above [marked in red]. There are plain lactose sugar structures that are similar to the Apis, but they are not as smooth. Also, a lot of the sugar chunks are larger than the Apis pieces.

Observational Findings for Apis mellifica 1M

Apis mellifica 1M Remedy

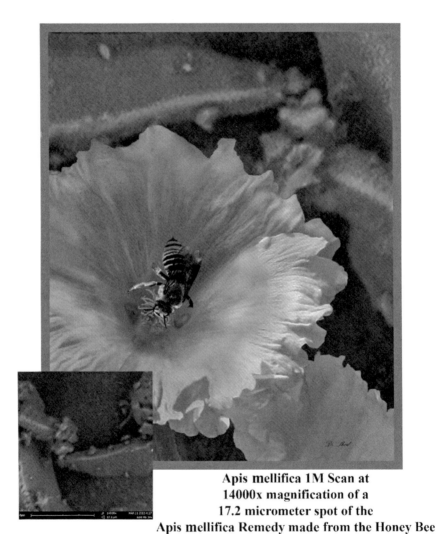

Apis mellifica 1M Scan at
14000x magnification of a
17.2 micrometer spot of the
Apis mellifica Remedy made from the Honey Bee

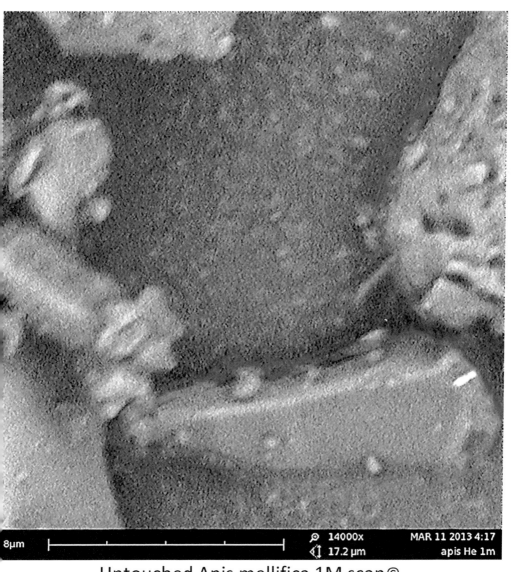

8µm   14000x   MAR 11 2013 4:17
    17.2 µm   apis He 1m

Untouched Apis mellifica 1M scan©

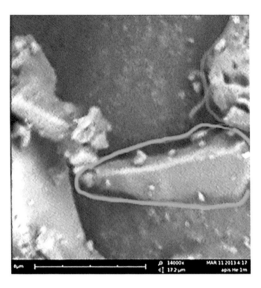

Apis mellifica 1M scan ©

This Apis mellifica 1M scan has the same tip-like structure as the Apis 6x scan. This structure is outlined in green. The piece is smooth with rounded edges and does not have any crevices. The structure in the above right-hand corner of the scan, which is marked in red, has crevices that are similar to the sugar pieces of the plain sugar scans. This piece of the Apis remedy seemed to be combined with the alcohol/water base properties to form one structure—an Apis/Alcohol/Water structure. The alcohol and the succussion process seem to have facilitated in forming an extraction of the remedy at the 1M concentration with its base solution. All the pictured scans of the Apis seem to show that this has occurred. These results seem to again suggest that a physiochemical extraction resulting from the alcohol/water liquid and the succussion with the Apis is forming this solution. The solution then separates the Apis structures within it to form the pieces that are shown in the scans. This probably occurs due to succussion process. This suggests that at each dilution level the alcohol and succussion are causing a change in the whole remedy/alcohol/water solution and the pieces that are formed. The process of the substance on each new level was started from the last level [one would use some of the 6x liquid to form the next level and so on]. This previously used substance is diluted again with alcohol/water, and then succussed again to form a new substance made up of the Apis remedy and the alcohol/water base.

The Apis remedy scans do not seem to mix with the sugar to which it is applied. These sugar formations, which still have their own characteristics, are found separate from the Apis/alcohol/water type pieces.

Arnica Montana 30c Remedy

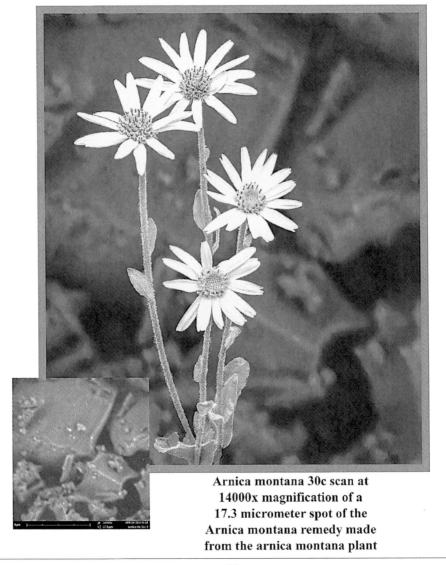

Arnica montana 30c scan at
14000x magnification of a
17.3 micrometer spot of the
Arnica montana remedy made
from the arnica montana plant

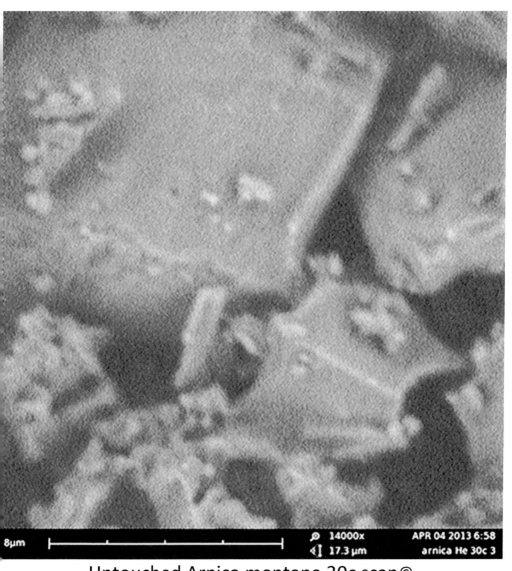

Untouched Arnica montana 30c scan©

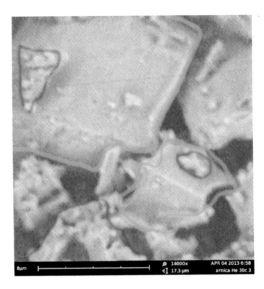

Arnica montana 30c scan©

As you can see from the scan pictured, the Arnica montana 30c [Arnica] has a similar surface to the Apis mellifica scans. Both show the smoothness that is like the smoothness of the alcohol/water base scans. Arnica pieces have bulky, angular, obtrusive shapes. Some shapes seem even like mountain boulders, which is curious since the flowers grow in the mountains. These shapes are different than the Apis scans and the base scans. The shapes are of various sizes, from being large structures to smaller ones. These types of shapes are a difference seen in all of the Arnica scans as a detail that is specific to Arnica. There are very few crevices in the Arnica structures. The pieces on the bottom left of the scan might be sugar, as well as the pieces outlined in red that are attached to the Arnica piece.

Arnica montana 1M Remedy

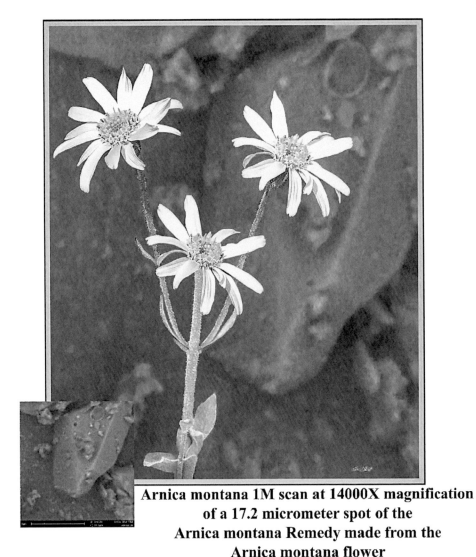

Arnica montana 1M scan at 14000X magnification
of a 17.2 micrometer spot of the
Arnica montana Remedy made from the
Arnica montana flower

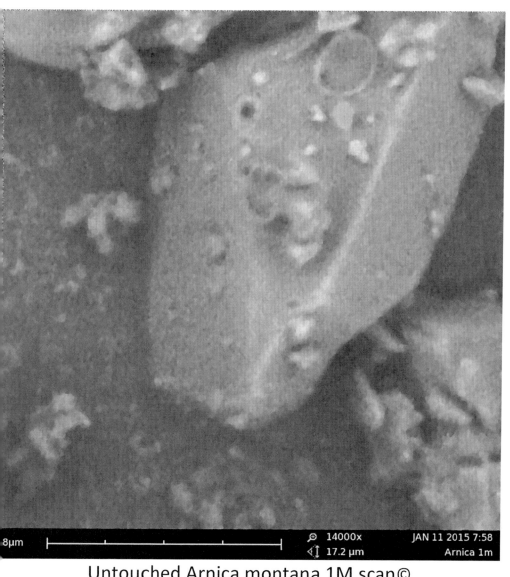

Untouched Arnica montana 1M scan©

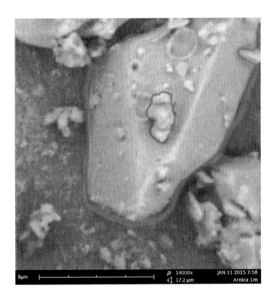

Arnica montana 1M scan©

The Arnica montana 1M scan shows the same chunky, angular type piece as the Arnica montana 30c scans. This piece is outlined in green. The small attached portions, which are outlined in red, are of another substance. The attachment of pieces to the Arnica chunks might suggest that the Arnica has a stickiness to its pieces. Also, there is one pockmark type crevice and a few shallow crevices in the Arnica 1M scan. This shows a slight mixing of the Arnica solution with the sugar.

All the Arnica scans observed seem to show a physiochemical mixing with the alcohol/water base into one whole solution.

This solution shows up in all the pieces, even in the pieces that are of a 1M potency.

Chamomilla 6x Remedy

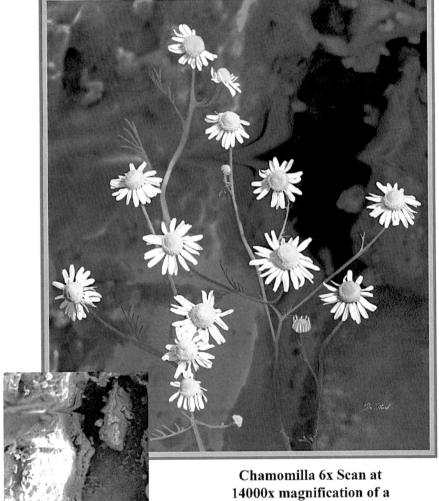

Chamomilla 6x Scan at
14000x magnification of a
17.2 micrometer spot of a
Chamomilla Remedy made from Chamomile

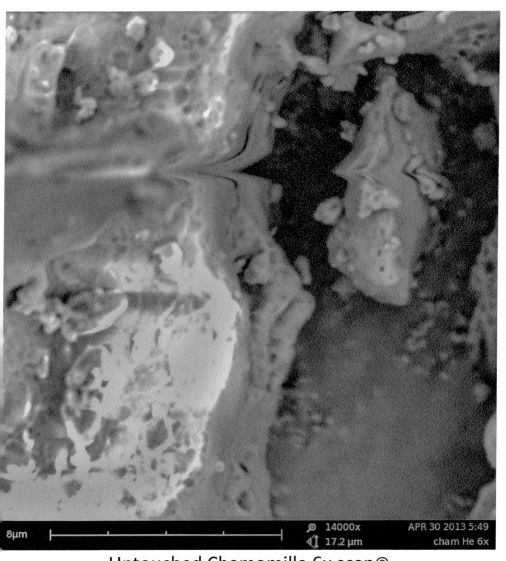

8µm | 14000x | APR 30 2013 5:49
17.2 µm | cham He 6x

Untouched Chamomilla 6x scan©

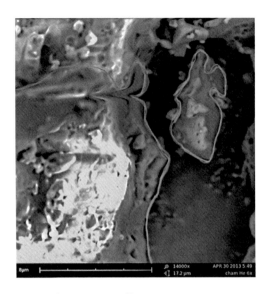

Chamomilla 6x scan©

All the Chamomilla remedy scans seem to be softer than the other remedies. They even seem to be softer than the lactose sugar powder used in this study. The Chamomilla was so soft it was difficult not to flatten out the sample to the point that a lot of the scans were very light, white, non-defined spots or even blown out parts. [The term 'blown out' is used in photography where the camera does not read the pixels in that particular area. Thus the pixels are blown out of the picture, or in this case the pictures of the scans.] The brighter the scans show up in the microscope, the more the areas of the scan have a blown-out part. The lower left side of the above scan has blown out areas. Many of the Chamomilla scans did have parts of the picture that were very bright or blown out. They also had parts that consistently looked smooth and bright, but not blown out, and had bumpy, lightened edges. The piece circled in green in the upper right of the scan above is a chunk that is like this.

Parts of the Chamomilla scanned pieces even look as though they have been ironed until they are totally smooth. Yet the pieces of Chamomilla have clear cut structures. They are not undefined, like a lot of the alcohol/water base scans. Both the base and the Chamomilla scans do contain smooth areas, but the Chamomilla pieces are lighter, and brighter than the alcohol/water base scans. This may be because the Chamomilla structures look smoother than the plain alcohol/water base scans.

There are crevices in the Chamomilla scans also, as the Chamomilla 6x scan shows. These crevices are shallow with smoothed edges, which is a difference that is particular to this remedy. The Chamomilla 6x crevices are like the sugar ones, but are softer and brighter than the sugar marks. One can see in the Chamomilla 6x scan above the brightness, and the softness. The parts of the pieces marked in green look very smooth and bright.

Observational Findings for Chamomilla 1M

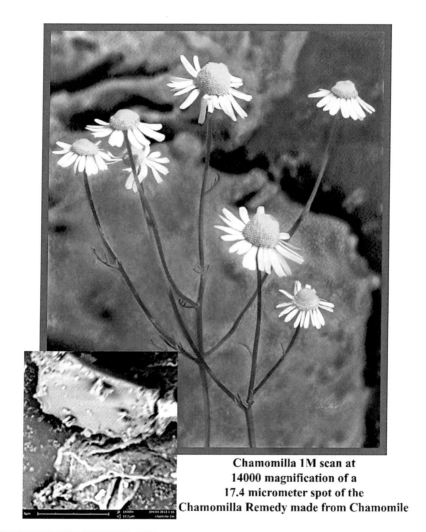

Chamomilla 1M Remedy

Chamomilla 1M scan at
14000 magnification of a
17.4 micrometer spot of the
Chamomilla Remedy made from Chamomile

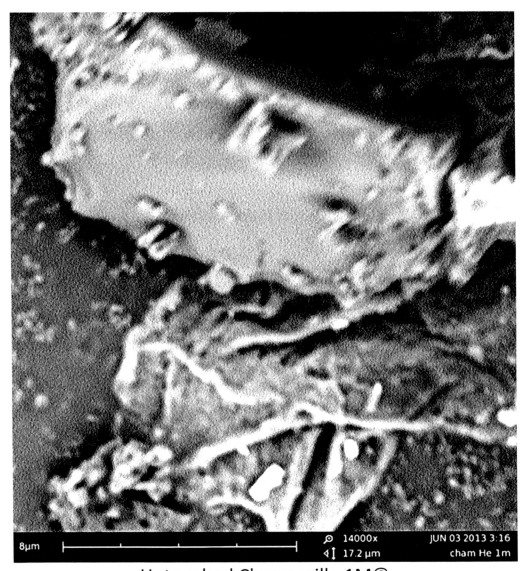

Untouched Chamomilla 1M©

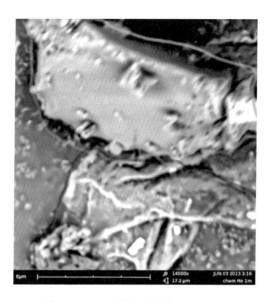

Chamomilla 1M scan©

The Chamomilla 1M scan above also shows the smooth, bright areas, as did the other Chamomilla scans on all levels of potencies, from a 6x to the 1M remedies that were observed. The bumps seen that are attached particles that are probably of another substance, such as the sugar lactose pieces. This might indicate a stickiness to the Chamomilla pieces. The chunk on the lower left hand side of the scan is probably another substance also. It is unknown what this substance might be. As with all the remedy scans, the Chamomilla scans show the smoothing as if there is a physiochemical mixing of properties of the alcohol/water base and the Chamomilla remedy to form one structure made of Chamomilla, alcohol and water.

Gelsemium sempervirens 200c Remedy

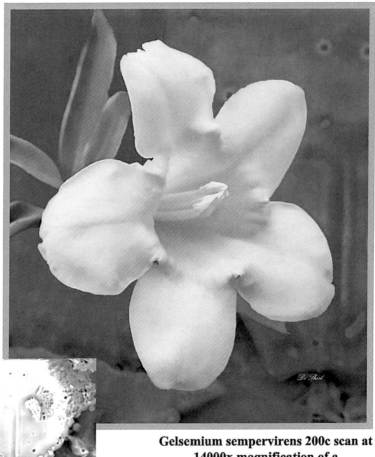

Gelsemium sempervirens 200c scan at
14000x magnification of a
17.2 micrometer spot of the
Gelsemium sempervirens Remedy made from
the Yellow Jessimine plant

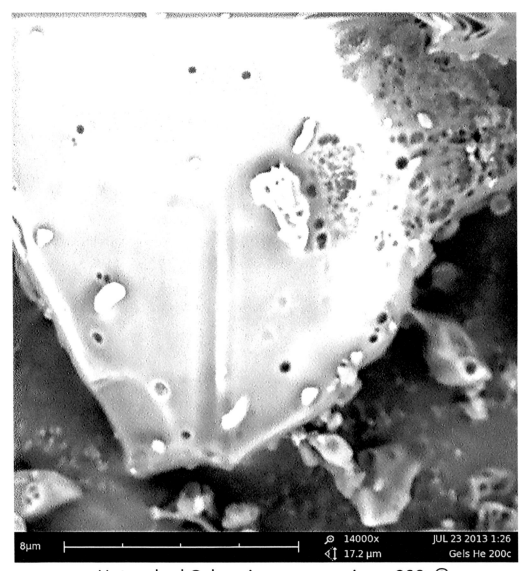

Untouched Gelsemium sempervirens 200c©

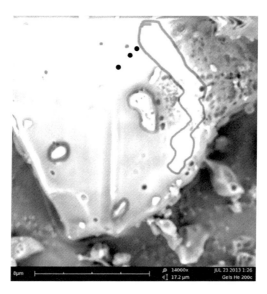

Gelsemium sempervirens 200c scan©

The Gelsemium Sempervirens [Gelsemium] scan has a smooth bright side like the Chamomilla, but it is not soft and sticky. Yet there were some areas of the Gelsemium scanned pictures that have blown out areas [circled in purple], which does seem to show a softness to that area. The Gelsemium does have more defined edges. Yet the Chamomilla remedy powders were difficult to work with due to their softness. This was not the case with the Gelsemium remedy powder. And, even those soft, blown out areas in the Gelsemium scans are not as distorted, and probably not as soft, as those in the Chamomilla scans. The Gelsemium scans also have a side that has distinct crevices with crisp edges, which the Chamomilla does not have. These crevices are shown in the upper right of the Gelsemium 200c's scan, which is the part that is marked by the green outline. These crevices are not throughout as it is with the plain lactose sugar scans. The Gelsemium scan almost looks as if it has a smoothed out area or a depressed area where some of the bumps are pressed down. These smoothed out areas are the brighter parts of the structures. The smoothness of the Gelsemium can be compared to the alcohol/water base scans, yet there are particular properties that seem to be from the Gelsemium remedy, such as the creviced sides and defined structures. The defined, creviced shapes are aspect of the Gelsemium scans which are different than the alcohol/water scans. The 200c scan of Gelsemium shown here has the properties discussed in this observation. These observed properties show up in most of the Gelsemium scans on all potency levels that were examined.

Gelsemium sempervirens 6x Remedy

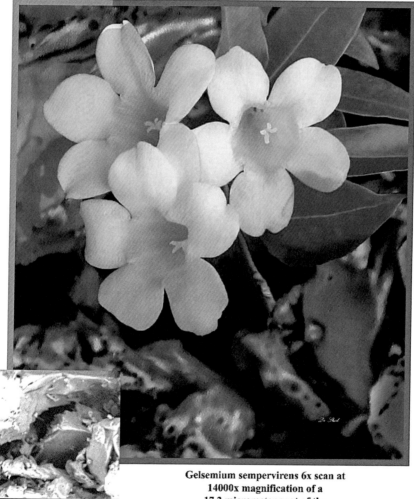

Gelsemium sempervirens 6x scan at
14000x magnification of a
17.2 micrometer spot of the
Gelsemium sempervirens Remedy made from the
Yellow Jessamine plant

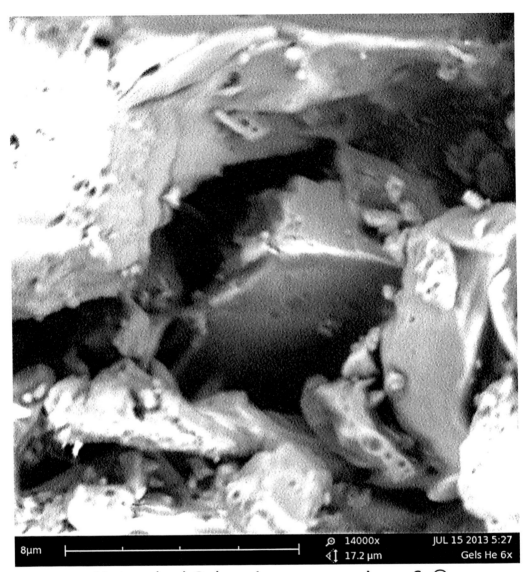

| 8μm | | 🔍 14000x | JUL 15 2013 5:27 |
| | | ⬍ 17.2 μm | Gels He 6x |

Untouched Gelsemium sempervirens 6x©

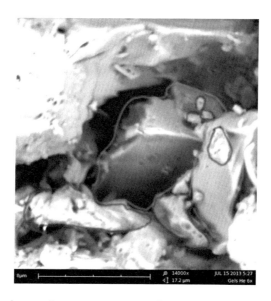

Gelsemium sempervirens 6x scan©

The Gelsemium 6x scan shown above has the same smooth, bright sides to the remedy chunks, some of which are marked in green. There are several pieces in the scan that are probably other substances, such as the lactose particles and insert substances [circled in red]. The upper left hand corner and a smaller area in the lower right side of this 6x scan are blown out areas, because they were too bright for the microscope to pick up those pixels. This is similar to the Chamomilla scans, except that the Gelsemium was not as soft to work with as the Chamomilla. The Gelsemium scan pictures probably have blown out areas due to their being ultra-smooth in that area, as with some of the Chamomilla. All the Gelsemium scans show similar properties, which indicates there is a similarity of traits in all the Gelsemium scans. Also all the Gelsemium scans show the same chemical mixture of the properties of Gelsemium combined with those of the alcohol/water base to form one particular structure for each piece of the Gelsemium/alcohol/water remedy.

Lachesis muta 6x Remedy

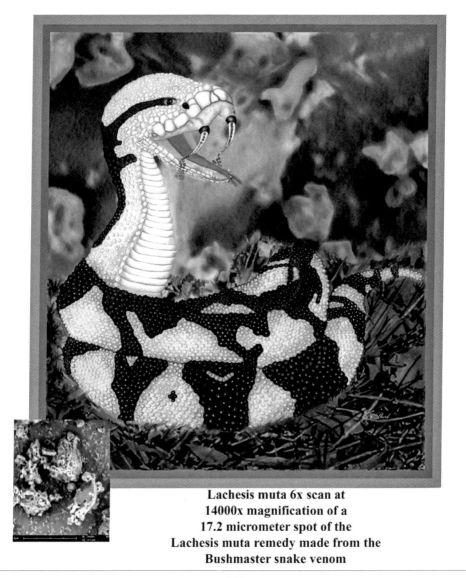

Lachesis muta 6x scan at
14000x magnification of a
17.2 micrometer spot of the
Lachesis muta remedy made from the
Bushmaster snake venom

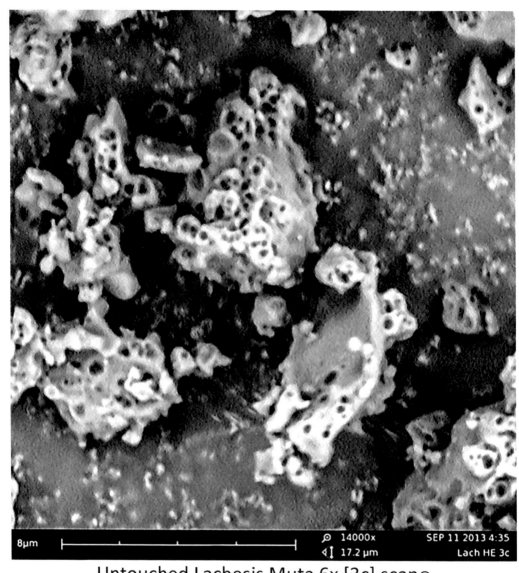

8μm   🔍 14000x   SEP 11 2013 4:35
◁↕ 17.2 μm   Lach HE 3c

Untouched Lachesis Muta 6x [3c] scan©

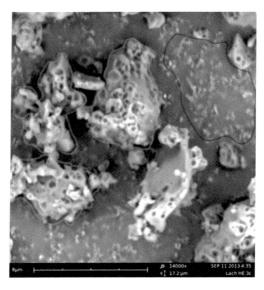

Lachesis mutus 6x [3c] scan©

The Lachesis mutus [Lachesis] sample, which comes from a homeopathic pharmacy in Great Britain[3] is a 3c; but that is the same potency level, with the same amount of processing, as the 6x remedies. For the sake of being uniform with the study, this Lachesis mutus remedy with be called a 6x.

This Lachesis scan, seen above, has pockmarks, as does the Gelsemium scan. But a lot of the Lachesis marks are larger and protruding, as if they are erupting. The whole structure looks a little bit rougher, and more lively with very marked eruptions. The marks are even larger and more protruding than the marks found in the base lactose sugar scans. There are still some plain sugar pieces which have regular looking crevices in the Lachesis scans.

There are some formations in the Lachesis scans that have larger, smoother areas than the base sugar scans. These Lachesis pieces are different from the eruptive ones. They are a second type of Lachesis structure. These secondary pieces are definitely defined and not flattened out as one large formation, which is in contrast to what the alcohol/water base scans showed. The pieces marked in green show the eruptive marks clearly. All of the lively eruptive pieces and the smoother structures throughout the all Lachesis scan group, which is all the scans in all the different potencies, show the same similar characteristic. All the other remedies scans have shown that they have similar traits within their groups also.

There are, as always, other substances shown in the scan, like the inert carbon background [marked in red]. The erupting, rougher structures and some smoother pieces are found in all the levels of the Lachesis scans, from the 6x to the 1M.

Lachesis muta 200c Remedy

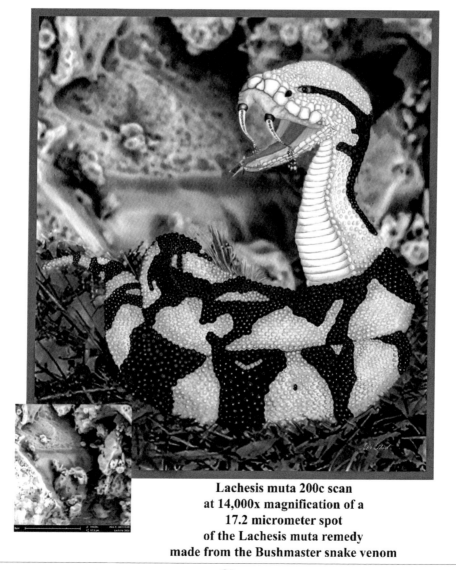

Lachesis muta 200c scan
at 14,000x magnification of a
17.2 micrometer spot
of the Lachesis muta remedy
made from the Bushmaster snake venom

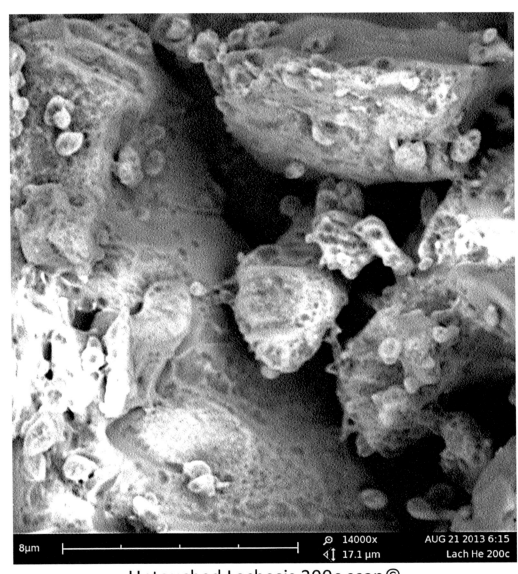

8µm | 14000x | AUG 21 2013 6:15
17.1 µm | Lach He 200c

Untouched Lachesis 200c scan©

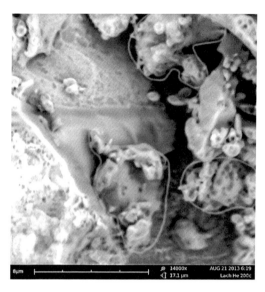

Lachesis mutus 200c scan©

Above is an example of the Lachesis mutus 200c scan shows the same properties as the Lachesis 6x scan, and all the Lachesis scans. Some of the Lachesis chunks are flatter and smoother than others. And there are some that have the pockmarks that are large and stick up more than the marks of the other remedies and the base sugar scans. As with all the remedies, there are some pieces that are an unknown type of formation. These pieces might be other impurities not identified in this study, such as the large structure in the left of the above scan. The surface of this piece is not the same as what seems to be the Lachesis chunks or the sugar pieces. The rough edge has different qualities also.

The alcohol/water smoothing properties showing in the Lachesis scans are seen in smoother structures and to lesser amounts in the rough, eruptive pieces. The Lachesis remedy seems to be reacting to the mixing of the alcohol/water and to the succussion differently than the other remedies, since there are two defined structures which are formed. The Lachesis extracted solution that is applied to the base sugar might also be reacting differently to the sugar. This is probably due to the inherent nature of the Lachesis mother tincture.

In the smoother Lachesis pieces the alcohol/water properties are very evident. The physiochemical solution of the Lachesis remedy can be detected in these structures in the Lachesis scans quite clearly. This physiochemical reaction is also occurring in the eruptive pockmarked piece, since it can be seen in the smoothness between these marks.

Medorrhinum 1M

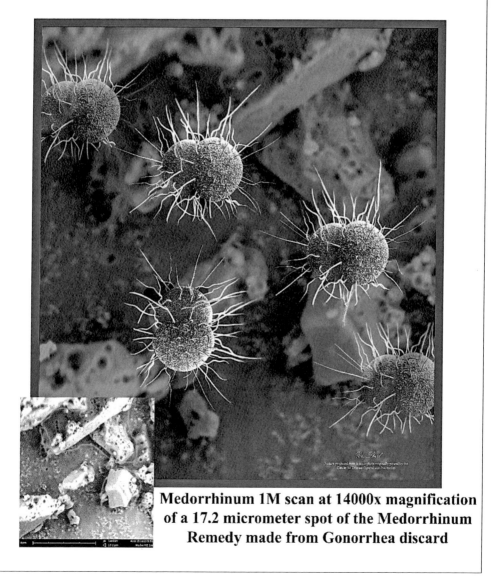

Medorrhinum 1M scan at 14000x magnification of a 17.2 micrometer spot of the Medorrhinum Remedy made from Gonorrhea discard

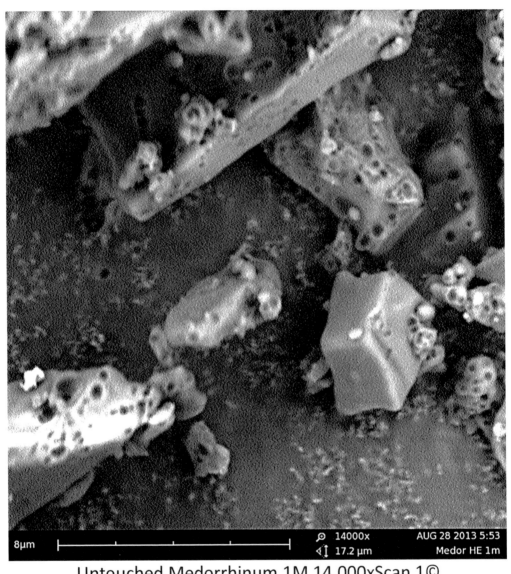

Untouched Medorrhinum 1M 14,000xScan 1©

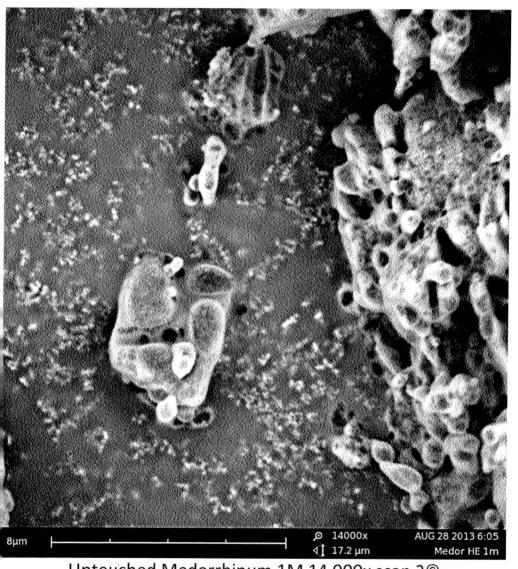

8μm 14000x AUG 28 2013 6:05
17.2 μm Medor HE 1m

Untouched Medorrhinum 1M 14,000x scan 2©

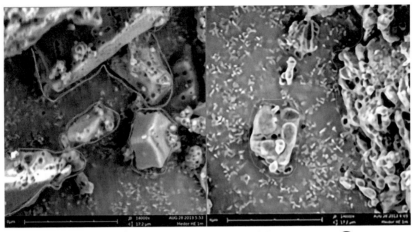

Medorrhinum 1M 14,000x scans ©

The Medorrhinum 1M scan has what seems to be hard

chunks that have remained somewhat intact, even after all

the processing this remedy has went through to reach the

1M level. They are similar to the Arnica chunks, yet the

Medorrhinum structures seem smaller, and a lot of the

structures are more abstract in shape than the Arnica pieces.

An example of this abstraction is in the shape of the structure

on the right of the scan on the left.

There are other Medorrhinum scans that seem to have a

breakdown of structures that results in a pronounced gritty-

like, rough surface and have little pieces stuck to the surface

that looked like broken glass. This collapse of the structures

can be seen more on a scan of 5000x magnification scans

rather than the 14,000x magnification scans. The greatly magnified 14,000x scan shows more of the details of this gritty type marks. In the 14,000x scan this surface seems to look like eruptive pockmarks, which is shown in the above scan on the right. These chunks that have very pronounced pockmarks look similar to the Lachesis scans. Both remedies have deep eruptive crevices. But the Medorrhinum's pockmarks are on various levels from their base piece, with some erupting from a higher point and some a lower point. The Lachesis marks are erupting more on one level. This can be seen in the picture of the Medorrhinum 1M scan on the right, above.

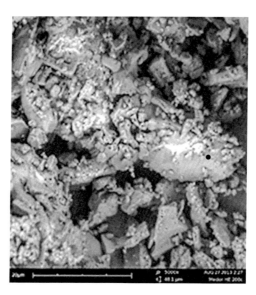

Medorrhinum 200c 5,000x scan©

Shown above is a picture of the 5,000x scan of Medorrhinum [and the untouched picture is shown next], which shows the texture of the whole surface. Medorrhinum has the gritty like pieces in the left-hand side of the scan, which is circled in green. This 5,000x scan It also has the smoother, angular, hard chunks, especially on the bottom and upper right part of the scan.

Note: The illustration photos of the gonorrhea are from a stock photo which was posted on the web and originally taken by the Center for Disease Control and Prevention.

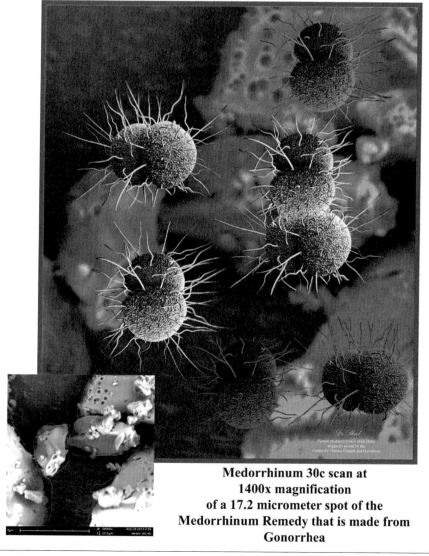

Medorrhinum 30c Remedy

Medorrhinum 30c scan at
1400x magnification
of a 17.2 micrometer spot of the
Medorrhinum Remedy that is made from
Gonorrhea

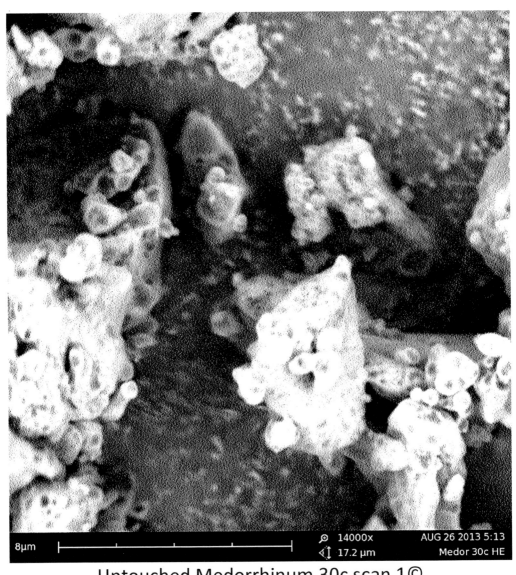

Untouched Medorrhinum 30c scan 1©

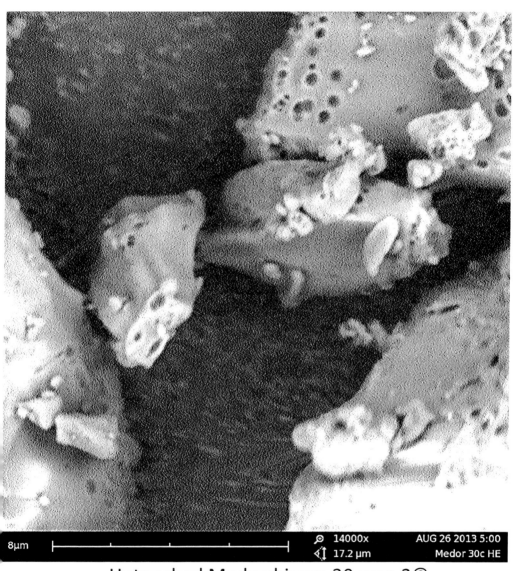

Untouched Medorrhinum 30 scan 2©

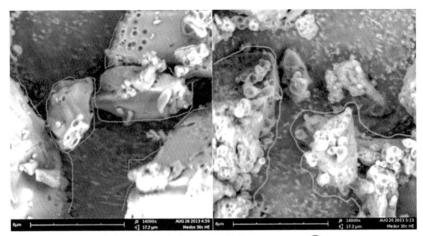

Medorrhinum 30c scans©

As can be seen in both the 30c and the 1M Medorrhinum scans, the smooth, delineated pieces have pockmarks which may be considered similar to the Gelsemium scans. The Gelsemium scans have marks that are fewer and spaced more apart than the marks seen in the Medorrhinum scan on the right. The Medorrhinum's chunky pieces that are similar to the Gelsemium pieces seem to have an overall smoothness. The shapes of the Medorrhinum chunks are different from the Gelsemium structures. The marks might be compared to the lactose sugar marks, but the general surface of the Medorrhinum pieces is smoother than the sugar. The Lachesis scans have similar eruptive type marks like the Medorrhinum scan above shown on the left. But the Lachesis marks seem to come from a more flat, smoother base on most of their pieces. Plus, a lot of the Lachesis pockmarks seem to be gathered near or on the end of the chunks. This second type of Medorrhinum piece has pockmarks that come from the base of the piece which is irregular and rough. Also the Medorrhinum pockmarks are spread out all over the pieces and are not gathered in any particular area.

These eruptive Medorrhinum marks might indicate, like the Lachesis, that the Medorrhinum interacts with the sugar in a more agitated way. The plain sugar scans do not show any roughness of their structure, nor do they show very eruptive crevices as the Medorrhinum scans show. Since both the Medorrhinum and the Lachesis have pieces that are smoother and some that are rough and eruptive, it is hard to tell why some of the remedies' solutions are showing these properties.

Although there are similarities between the different remedy scans, all the remedies have their particular aspects that make them unique. The Medorrhinum scans have areas that are broken down to a 'gritty like' surface with its hard pieces interspersed in this grit, which is seen clearly in the 5,000x scan that is pictured with the Medorrhinum 1M write up. The surfaces of the gritty pieces are rough and uneven, which makes the pockmarks vary in height. As already mentioned, there are also smoother formations. This characteristic is seen only in Medorrhinum and Lachesis scans groups.

The traits of eruptive structures, with their grittiness, were not seen at all in the alcohol/water base scans, nor in the sugar base scans. What reactions are occurring or not occurring with these pieces is unknown for now. But a guess could be ventured that this is a trait of the mother tincture, since the Medorrhinum nosode [which is what this type of remedy is called] is made from gonorrhea. The remedy [outside of this study] is used to treat people with the symptoms of gonorrhea that have a 'breakdown of their health', since they have lot of inflammation or irritation, and can have fever, chills, and so on. Remedies are picked, from the mother tincture on upward to the higher potencies, due to the similarities of their energy with the problems they are to treat. The problems the Medorrhinum' treats is similar to the properties of the eruptive structures since gonorrhea is very disruptive to a person, especially if left untreated. As we have seen, the smooth Medorrhinum pieces are totally different in their characteristics.

The smoothness of these chunky Medorrhinum structures can be contributed in part to the smoothing properties of the alcohol/water solution. But there does seem to be the same physiochemical mixing of the substances in some of the pieces of this remedy, the smoother ones.

Observational Findings for Natrum muriaticum 6x

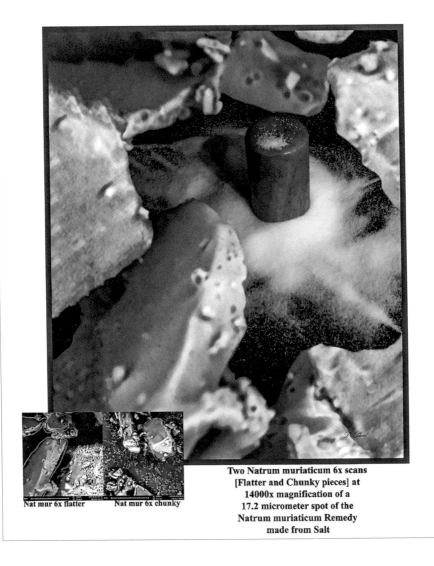

Natrum muriaticum 6x Remedy

Nat mur 6x flatter   Nat mur 6x chunky

Two Natrum muriaticum 6x scans
[Flatter and Chunky pieces] at
14000x magnification of a
17.2 micrometer spot of the
Natrum muriaticum Remedy
made from Salt

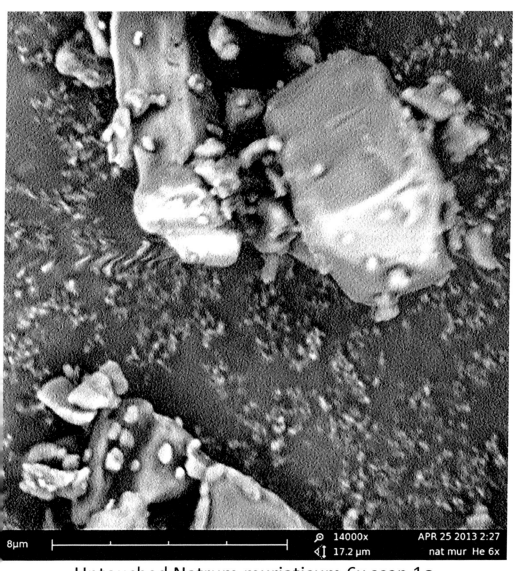

Untouched Natrum muriaticum 6x scan 1©

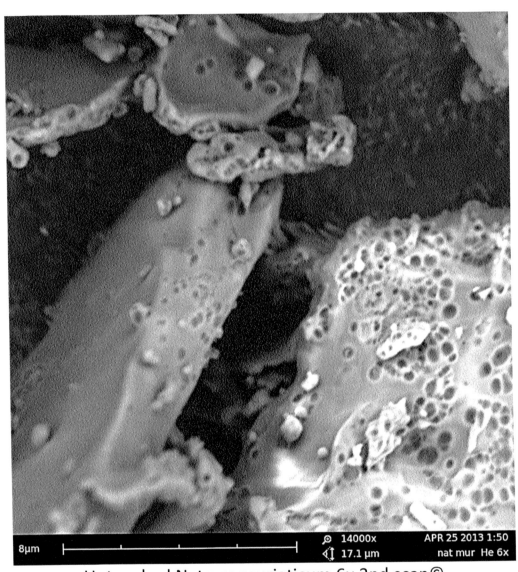

Untouched Natrum muriaticum 6x 2nd scan©

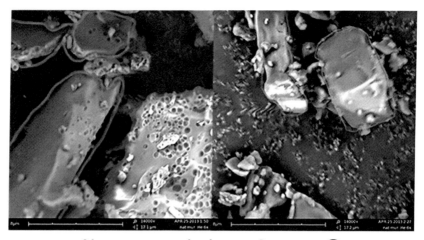

Natrum muriaticum 6x scans©

These two Natrum muriaticum 6x scans are shown to point out their two different features; the angular chunks and the flattened pieces. The Natrum muriaticum [Nat mur] 6x scan on the right has a lot of the chunkier pieces which have rounded edges of almost 45⁰ angles, on several of their sides. Some of these pieces are even similar to a cube or rectangular shape. The Medorrhinum scan had a piece that was similar to a cube, but that was the only one in that shape in all the Medorrhinum scans. A person could not come to the conclusion that this is a trait seen in the Medorrhinum scans. Whereas, in the Nat mur scans, there are many that have this angular shape. This shape is similar to the Arnica structures, but the Nat mur pieces are smaller than the Arnica ones.

Nat mur also has similar smoothed out, flatter pieces that are seen in several of the remedies, such as the Gelsemium. These are shown in the other Nat mur scans, shown in the left scan picture. This scan picture has pieces that look a bit flattened and deflated. These structures look similar in thickness to a pancake or a slice of bread, as seen in the three green marked structures.

Most of what seems to be the Nat mur chunks and slices have very few crevices; thus, the creviced structure, marked in red in the left scan, is probably not a Nat mur piece. It is probably a sugar piece. The defining aspects of the Nat mur seems to be their chunky or flattened pieces, which have few, or even, no pockmarks. There are unidentified chunks that are varied in shape in the right Nat mur scan that have a lot of smaller, non-creviced pieces attached to them. It is unknown whether these are different shapes of the Nat mur or other unidentified formations.

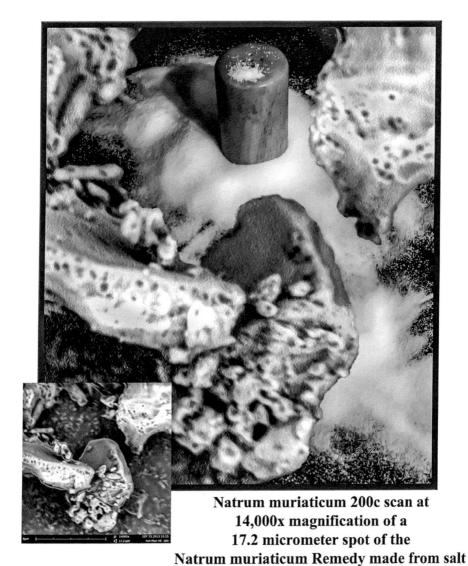

Natrum muriaticum 200c Remedy

Natrum muriaticum 200c scan at
14,000x magnification of a
17.2 micrometer spot of the
Natrum muriaticum Remedy made from salt

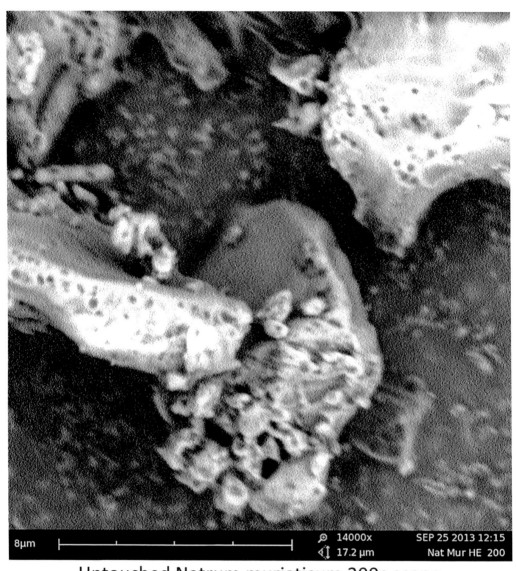

8μm 14000x SEP 25 2013 12:15
17.2 μm Nat Mur HE 200

Untouched Natrum muriaticum 200c scan©

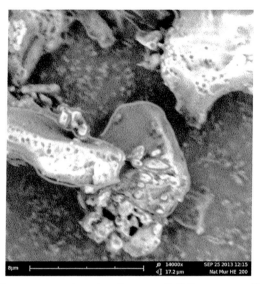

Natrum muriaticum 200c scan©

The Natrum muriaticum 200c scan shows the flattened structure with many attached pieces on the end of the structure, as can be seen marked in green with the attached pieces in red. The Nat mur flat, or chunky structures are seen in scans at every level of their potencies. The Nat mur slice is very smooth with pockmarks on the end of the it. This piece was probably affected by the alcohol/water solution.

Many of the pieces in all the Nat mur scans have several attached particles, like the one shown in the area outlined in red in the 200c scan. The Nat mur scans might have a smooth stickiness of their structures that seems to attract other substances to attach to them in bulk. In this Nat mur 200c scan, the attached pieces might be lactose sugar particles. As with all the scans of all the remedies, there seems to be a physiochemical mixing of the substances of Nat mur and the alcohol/water solution shown by the smoothing property of the alcohol/water solution. The alcohol does this by changing the solution into an extraction because the alcohol is a solvent. Then the succussion's pounding and shaking would finish the process by extracting, or separating the homeopathic particles in the solution and thus creating a new extracted solution.

Observational Findings for Ruta graveolens 1M

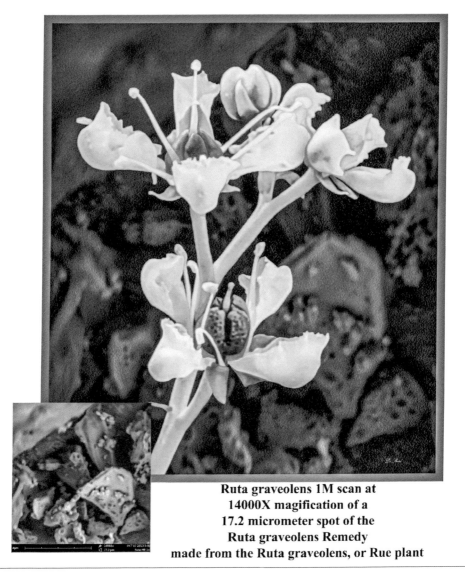

Ruta graveolens 1M Remedy

Ruta graveolens 1M scan at
14000X magification of a
17.2 micrometer spot of the
Ruta graveolens Remedy
made from the Ruta graveolens, or Rue plant

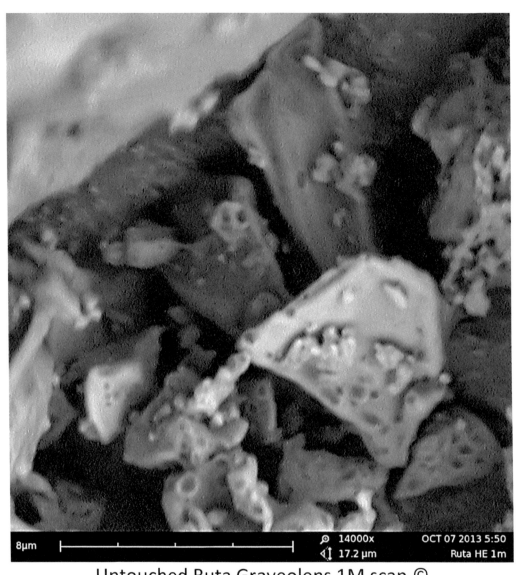

8µm   14000x   OCT 07 2013 5:50
17.2 µm   Ruta HE 1m

Untouched Ruta Graveolens 1M scan ©

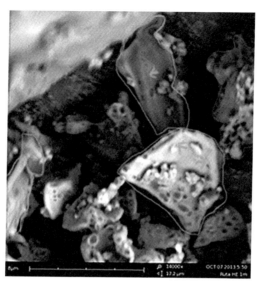

Ruta graveolens 1M scan©

The Ruta graveolens [Ruta] 1M scan shows structures that are smooth, like many of the other scans of the remedy. But the Ruta scan has edges that have rims on them, as pointed out by the green arrows. There are pieces of other substances attached to these rimmed chunks. These attached pieces are similar the ones found in the Nat mur scans. But these pieces are fewer in number and are located in various places on the Ruta scan. Only a few crevices are on the rimmed structures of the Ruta scans, which is similar to some of the scans of other remedies, such as the Nat mur or the Gelsemium scans. The ridge formations are seen on both potencies of the Ruta scans and are particular to the group of

Ruta scans. These ridges are not found on any of the other scans of any of the other remedies that were studied.

Observational Findings for Ruta graveolens 30c

Ruta graveolens 30c Remedy

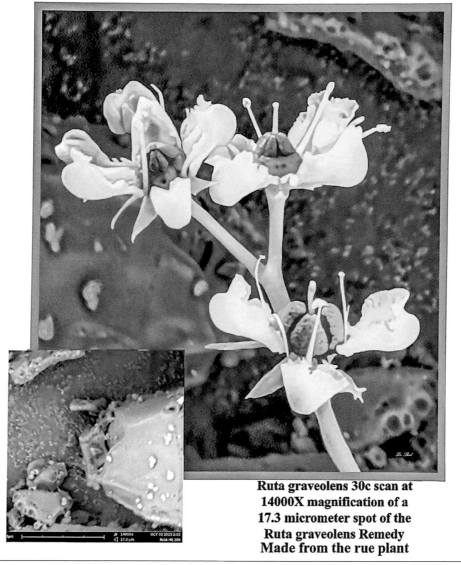

Ruta graveolens 30c scan at
14000X magnification of a
17.3 micrometer spot of the
Ruta graveolens Remedy
Made from the rue plant

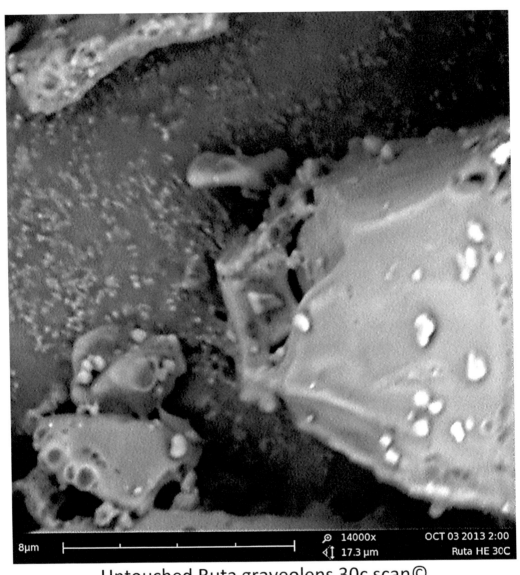

Untouched Ruta graveolens 30c scan©

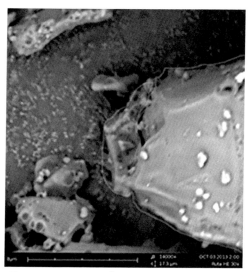
Ruta graveolens 30c scan©

The Ruta graveolens 30c scan, shown above, has two ridges that are shown as lighter marks [also pointed out with small green arrows] on the top of the larger piece on the right of the scan. The light edge around the left and bottom side of this same structure would also be indicative of a rim. This type of rim formation looks similar to the ends of some bones [See below the picture of a bone], which is a part of the body that Ruta helps. Ruta particularly helps when there is bruising to the covering of the bone, or the periosteum. There are very few small crevices on the pieces in the 30c scan. The formations in this Ruta scan do have smoothed surfaces like the smoothness found in the alcohol/water base scans. But the alcohol/water base scans, as previously stated, do not have the defined, structures. Nor do they have rimmed edges. One can conclude that the same physiochemical changes have occurred with the group of Ruta scans.

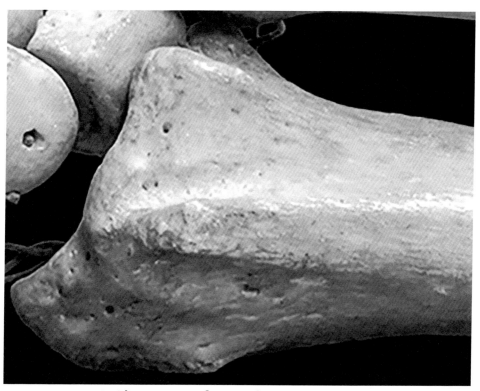

A Close-up of a Radius Arm Bone,
which is from a stock photo posted to the web

Observational Findings for Sepia 200c

Sepia 200c Remedy

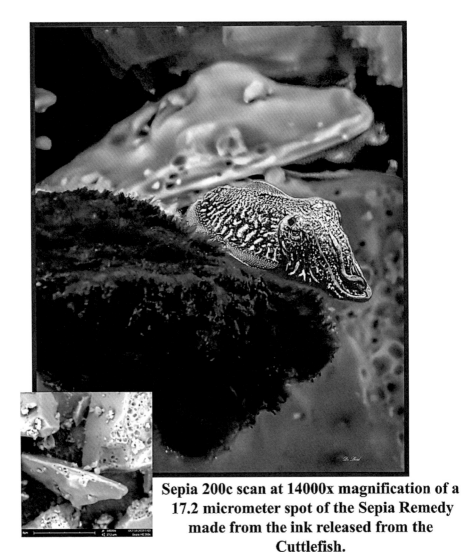

Sepia 200c scan at 14000x magnification of a 17.2 micrometer spot of the Sepia Remedy made from the ink released from the Cuttlefish.

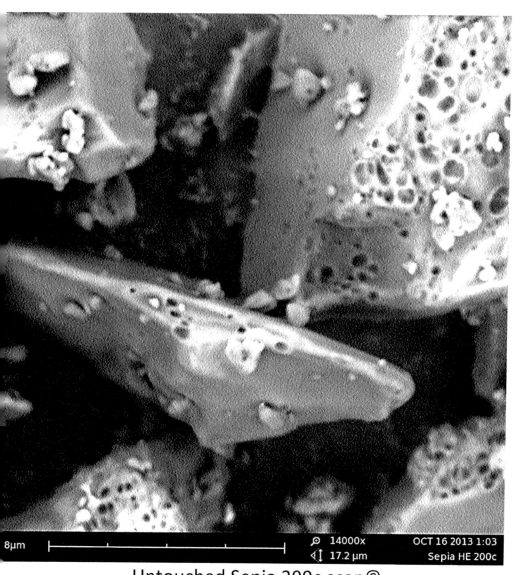

| 8µm | | | | | ⊘ 14000x | OCT 16 2013 1:03 |
| | | | | | ⬍ 17.2 µm | Sepia HE 200c |

Untouched Sepia 200c scan©

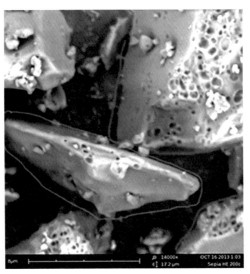

Sepia 200c scan©

The Sepia 200c scan seems to show the crevices in clusters spread throughout the structures, often on one side. There are chunks of various sizes in the Sepia scans. But some of the Sepia pieces are flattened, almost dish shaped in appearance. Strangely, these flattened pieces look similar to the flattened out cuttlefish, when it is swimming away and releasing its ink. The Sepia remedy is made from ink that the cuttlefish projects. The comparison of the shape of the Sepia remedy piece with the cuttlefish can be seen in the illustration for the Sepia 200c remedy, which was shown previously at the beginning of the chapter. Other remedies had pieces that looked flattened, such as the Lachesis scans, but they were not as smooth as the pieces in the Sepia scans. Gelsemium scans had smooth flattened structures with crevices on some of the sides of some of their pieces, but they were brighter than the Sepia formations. Plus the Gelsemium scans had some random deeper crevices within the smooth areas, than the Sepia does. The shapes, markings, and areas of smoothness seen in the Sepia scans seem particular to the Sepia remedy. Some of the smoothness seen on the Sepia structures, as seen in almost all the remedy scans, is probably the effect of the alcohol/water base mixing with the Sepia. The changes to the solution are then finished with the succussion process.

Sepia 6x Remedy

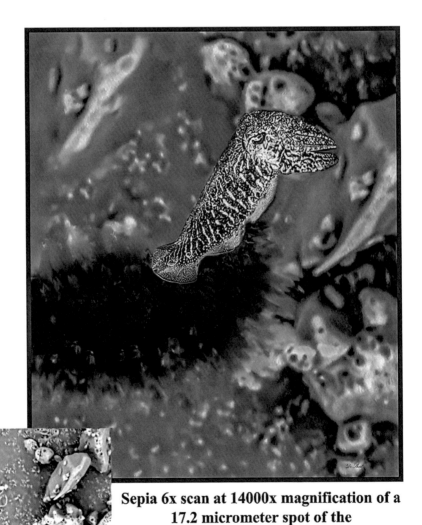

Sepia 6x scan at 14000x magnification of a 17.2 micrometer spot of the Sepia Remedy made from the Ink released from the Cuttlefish

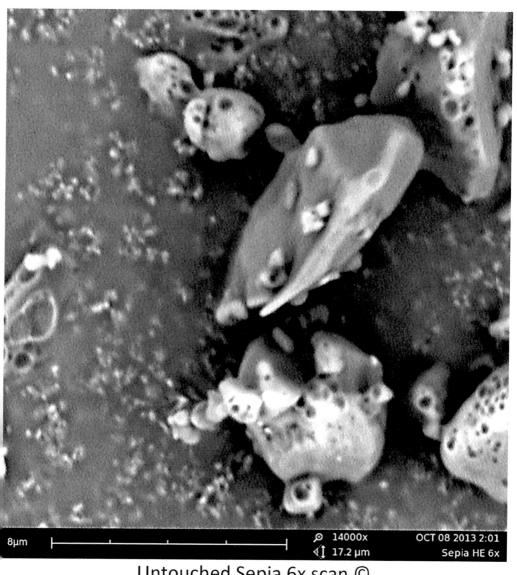

8µm   14000x   OCT 08 2013 2:01
17.2 µm   Sepia HE 6x

Untouched Sepia 6x scan ©

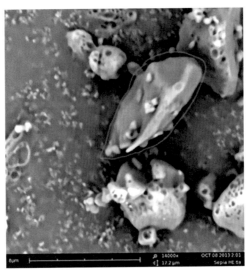

Sepia 6x scan©

The Sepia 6x scan, seen above, clearly shows a smooth, disc shaped structure. The two other pieces also show the chunky Sepia structures. There seems to be fewer pock marks in the Sepia 6x scan than in the 200c scan, but the marks that are there are in clusters. All the Sepia scans have clearly defined, smooth formations with distinctive edges, which were probably formed due to the succussion process. One can see the same smoothing of the surface found on the Sepia pieces, which probably occurred due to the effect of the alcohol. Thus, there were probably physiochemical changes of the substances in the 6x Sepia scan, as there were with the other remedies.

Observational Findings for Sulfur 30c

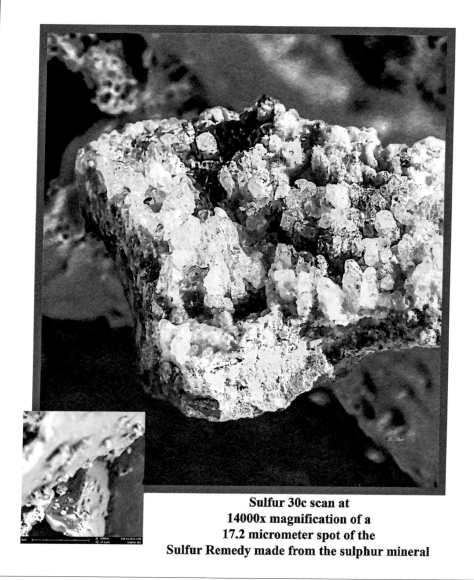

Sulfur 30c Remedy

Sulfur 30c scan at
14000x magnification of a
17.2 micrometer spot of the
Sulfur Remedy made from the sulphur mineral

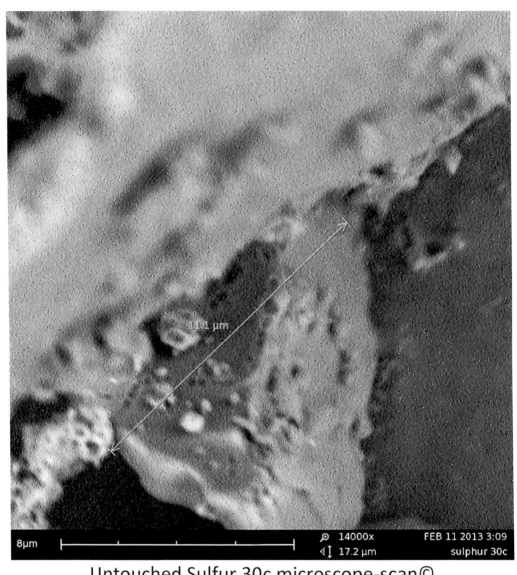

Untouched Sulfur 30c microscope-scan©

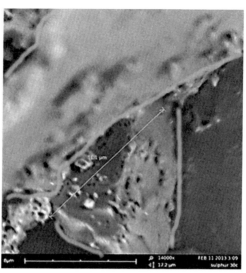

Sulfur 30c scan©

This Sulfur spelling is used because it is seen in scientific text with this spelling. Other texts use Sulphur as the spelling for this remedy. Sulfur 30c scan, as seen above, was measured within the microscope. This was done because many of the Sulfur scans had very large pieces, even though a small amount of pieces were not large. The large Sulfur piece measured here is 11.1μm. This measurement seems to be of only the tip of this structure. The other piece in this scan is even larger. The Sulfur structure is so large it is blurred because the microscope camera could not get the piece in focus at 14,000x magnification.

The structures of the Sulfur scans do not seem to have any particular shape, even though they are all well-defined pieces. A lot of them have some attached little chunks, and some crevices. But these crevices are in various places on the pieces. There seems to be a lot of variety of the shapes and the marks in the Sulfur scans, but most have some smoothness. This smoothness probably comes from the physiochemical reaction of the Sulfur with the alcohol/water base. There are formations of Sulfur, though, that have very rough surfaces, similar to the Medorrhinum or Lachesis. And there were other similarities to the other remedy scans also. There were a few smaller pieces that were found in the scan of the Sulfur remedy. These pieces seem specifically to have traits that are like other remedies, such as smooth angular edges on the chunk.

It would seem that the particular characteristic of Sulfur is that most of the pieces are large in size and that it has, mostly, two different surfaces to the well-defined formations. The rough surfaced chunks were too rough to be sugar pieces. But there definitely were other structures that were sugar pieces that were found in and among the Sulfur scans, as there were with all the remedies.

The essence, or nature of the Sulphur remedy [not the scans] is that it is a polycrest. This remedy has many uses and treats many things. There is a lot of variety in what this remedy does.

This essence seems to match the way the Sulfur scans are in that they, too, have a lot of variety in their shapes, size and texture. Yet none of the piece found were like the base scans of alcohol/water or sugar.

Observational Findings for Sulfur 1M

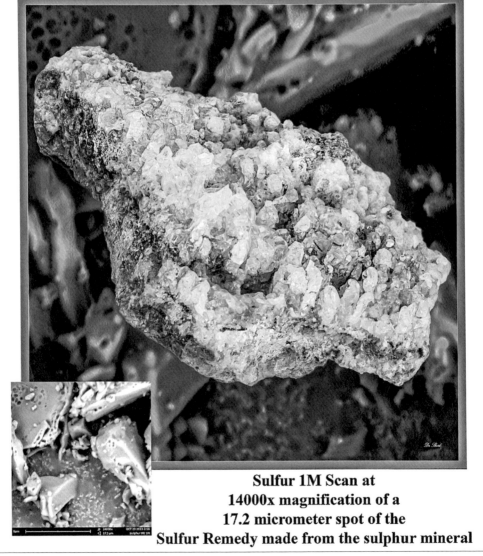

Sulfur 1M Remedy

Sulfur 1M Scan at 14000x magnification of a 17.2 micrometer spot of the Sulfur Remedy made from the sulphur mineral

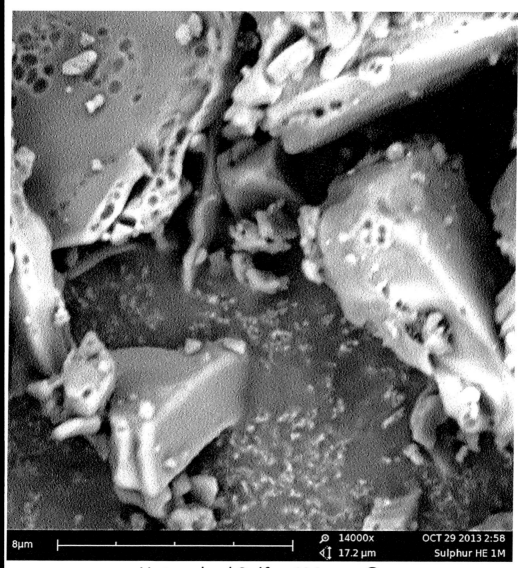

8μm | | | | | | 🔎 14000x · OCT 29 2013 2:58
⬍ 17.2 μm · Sulphur HE 1M

Untouched Sulfur 1M scan©

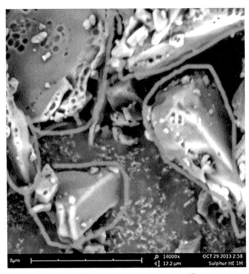

Sulfur 1M scans©

The left Sulfur 1M scan clearly shows the variety of shapes

and placements of crevices. And three of these five

structures are too large to fit into this scan. All the remedies

used in this study had some variety of shape and size. But

Sulfur had more variety than the other remedies. There were

Sulfur pieces in other scans that seemed to be too large to be

to be captured with the 14,000x magnification setting of the

microscope. A lot of the scanned structures of Sulfur were

the largest of all the remedies scanned. Arnica had large

structures also, and there was a variety of chunky shapes. But

the Sulfur pieces were larger and not all chunky. Some were

flattened dish shaped pieces, as shown above on the left. Some had more crevices than the Arnica.

The physiochemical mixture of the Sulfur remedy with the alcohol/water base can be detected in the structures of the smooth pieces in the scans quite clearly. This physiochemical reaction most likely is occurring in the more marked pieces too, but it is not as evident. And, as previously stated, the succussion process seems to separate the extracted solution into defined categories of pieces.

Summary, Conclusions, Past Research, And References

Summary and Conclusions

In summary, particular features were found for each individual remedy in all the 10 remedies scanned, at all the potency levels scanned, which were 6x, 30c, 200c, and 1M. None of the remedies looked like the plain alcohol/water base scans. Yet all of the remedies did have some aspect of their features that were similar to the smoothing effect of the alcohol/water solution that was used to dilute the remedy in preparation for that potency level. This was probably due to the fact that the alcohol is a solvent. Due to observations regarding the alcohol/water, the theory was reached that there are changes occurring due to the alcohol used in the making of each level of the remedy's potency. The succussion process, which is also used in the making of the potency levels, would then increase the extraction procedure by helping to form separate homeopathic remedy pieces though the agitation of the pounding and shaking used in the succussion. This would complete the changes that are being made to the remedy.

These changes are physiochemical in nature since they alter the remedy chemistry and structures. The remedy/alcohol/water dilution causes the chemical change. Then the succussion causes the physical change of the structures.

All of the different remedies showed lactose sugar features in some parts of the scans collected from that particular remedy.

The effects of the lactose sugar were found in addition to the alcohol/water's smoothing effects. In some of the scans where the remedies were seen, the lactose particles were separate from the remedy formations. In other scans, the sugar seemed to be a part of those formations. The ones that were separate were sometimes attached to the outside of remedy structures. Then there were scans that showed mostly or almost all structures that looked like the lactose sugars and other unidentified pieces. Those scans might have homeopathic nanoparticles that this study could not observe. In conclusion, each remedy does have its own particular and distinguishable feature(s). And, these special features are viewed on all the levels of potencies of the remedy that were observed under the microscope's 14,000X magnification.

These unique features can be attributed to the substance as remaining pieces of remedy in spite of the various and many dilutions and succussions. The dilutions and succussions do seem to change the whole new potency level of substance into a new extracted solution.

Past Research

Past research has been done regarding the topic of this empirical study of homeopathic remedies that seem to support the theory formulated here. A few of these research studies are posted in PubMed [US National Library of Medicine, National Institutes of Health] are:

Variation in Fourier transform infrared spectra of some homeopathic potencies and their diluent media. This research was done by Sukul NC, Ghosh S, Sukul A, Sinhababu SP in 2005. Their conclusion was: "The potencies and their diluent media therefore differ from each other in the number of hydrogen-bonded water species and their hydrogen-bonding strength."[4]

The defining role of structure (including epitaxy) in the plausibility of homeopathy. This research was done by M. L. Rao, R. Roy, I. R. Bell, and R. Hoover in 2007. Their conclusion was, "Preliminary data obtained using Raman and Ultra-Violet-Visible (UV-VIS) spectroscopy illustrate the ability to distinguish two different homeopathic medicines (Nux vomica and Natrum muriaticum) from one another and to differentiate, within a given medicine, the 6c, 12c, and 30c potencies."[1]

Extreme homeopathic dilutions retain starting materials: A nanoparticulate perspective. This research was done by PS Chikramane, AK Suresh, JR Bellare, SG Kane in 2010. Their conclusion was: "Using market samples of metal-derived medicines from reputable manufacturers, we have demonstrated for the first time by Transmission Electron Microscopy (TEM), electron diffraction and chemical analysis by Inductively Coupled Plasma-Atomic Emission Spectroscopy (ICP-AES), the presence of physical entities in these extreme dilutions, in the form of nanoparticles of the starting metals and their aggregates."[5]

References

1. M. L. Rao, R. Roy, I. R. Bell, and R. Hoover, "The defining role of structure (including epitaxy) in the plausibility of homeopathy," Homeopathy, vol. 96, pp. 175–182, 2007. [PubMed post: PMID:17678814]

2. Samal S, Geckeler KE. "Unexpected solute aggregation in water on dilution." Chem Commun, 2001; 21: 2224–2225.

3. Helios Homoeopathy Ltd at: 89 - 97 Camden Rd, Tunbridge Wells, Kent TN1 2QR [UK]

4. NC Sukul, S Ghosh, A Sukul, SP Sinhababu, "Variation in Fourier transform infrared spectra of some homeopathic potencies and their diluent media," Journal of Alternative Complementary Medicine, vol.5, pp. 807-12, 2005. [PubMed post PMID:16296914]

5. PS Chikramane, AK Suresh, JR Bellare, SG Kane, "Extreme homeopathic dilutions retain starting materials: A

nanoparticulate perspective", Homeopathy, vol.4, pp 231-42, 2010 [PubMed post: PMID:20970092

Addendum

Addendum: The 'Foot Prints' of the Essence of the Scanned Remedies

What is termed here as the essence of the remedies seems to be the energy of the life force, or vital force, as Dr. Hahnemann called it, that permeated the original substance from which the remedies are made. These substances and their energies are carried through all the different potencies of homeopathic remedies by the processing of each of the remedies at each level of potency. This energy has left its footprint, which can be observed in the scans of the remedies. Here listed below are descriptions of what I believed to be the signs or footprints of the vital forces of the remedies. [Dr. Hahnemann is considered the founder of homeopathy.]

Apis mellifica [Made from the Honey Bee]- A lot of the Apis mellifica scanned pieces look like a swollen, flattened stinger. Part of the essence of the remedy is the stinging, swelling action that the remedy treats.

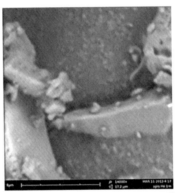

Apis mellifica 1M scan©

Arnica montana [Made from the Arnica montana flowering plant which grows in the mountainous areas] – Most of the Arnica montana scans look bulkier and angular, like mountain boulders, or large rocks. The remedy's footprint is that the structures seems to look like the boulders from the area where the plant grows.

Arnica's action is to mostly help with the bruises, mainly of muscles. It is a largely used remedy and is sold in bulk.

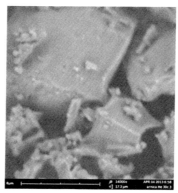

Arnica Montana 30c scan©

Chamomilla [Made from the Chamomile flowering plant]

The Chamomilla remedy powder used for the scans was a softer powder than the other remedies. It was so soft it was difficult not to flatten out the sample so much that it would make the scan was too light, like a bright white spot. Some of the Chamomilla scans consistently looked smooth and bright, with all the irritating edges lightened and softened. One of the remedy's actions is to smooth out the nervous, irritated feelings the person has and thus brighten their mood. This action fits the look and description of the Chamomilla scan pieces, and thus its essence.

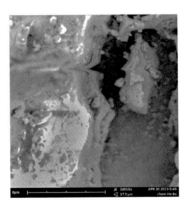

Chamomilla 6x scan©

Gelsemium sempervirens [Made from the Gelsemium, or Carolina Jessamine flowering plant] - The Gelsemium sempervirens scan almost looks as if it was smoothed out, or the bumps were depressed and the whole structure brightened. The remedy of Gelsemium interacts with the central nervous system when it is depressed, and sometimes paralyzed. Gelsemium helps to make you feel better, smoothing out your 'rough' feelings; thus, it makes you feel lighter. [The scan below seems to show a mark that looks like a part of a spine. This is not something that is part of all the Gelsemium scans, but just this one.] The Gelsemium scan visually looks like the action that the Gelsemium remedy performs, therefore, the Gelsemium scan pieces have an essence that matches their remedy's actions.

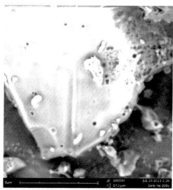

Gelsemium Sempervirens 200c ©

Lachesis muta [Made from the Bushmaster snake venom]

Some of the Lachesis muta scan look a bit rougher, and with more marked eruptions that seem to be bursting and very lively. The marks of Lachesis seem to protrude more than any of the other scans from the other remedies. These pieces match the remedy's action because the Lachesis remedy is for a person that hemorrhages, and has intense, eruptive emotions. The person that needs Lachesis might have emotions that are very suppressed but could erupt at any moment. This eruptive attribute seems to fit the essence of what the Lachesis scans look like.

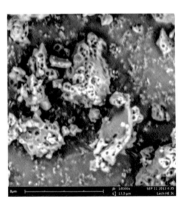

Lachesis Muta 6x ©

Medorrhinum [Made from the Neisseria gonorrhoeae bacteria]- Hard chunks were found in some of the Medorrhinum scans that had seemed to hold on to their structure and did not break down as much as the rest of the pieces in the scan. The rest of the scanned section seems to have a breakdown of their structures. This breakdown of structure can be seen more on a scan of 5,000x magnification than in the 14,000x magnification. The Medorrhinum remedy treats conditions that a person can be born with; thus, the problem would have started prior to their present life, such as an inherited problem that holds on in a family from generation to generation. This symptom matches the first part of the Medorrhinum scanned structures; the hard chunks that seem to have held on to their form. Medorrhinum also treats people who have a breakdown of their strength and constitutional health. This is seen in the second part of the Medorrhinum scans, where there is a breakdown of the pieces in the scanned remedy chunks. This indicates that the Medorrhinum scans show the essence of both parts of the remedy's actions.

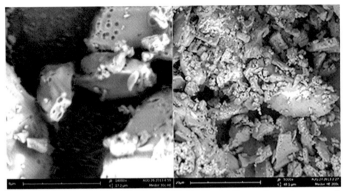

Medorrhinum 30c 14,000x © magnification is on the left and Medorrhinum 200c 5,000x magnification scan is on the right©

Natrum muriaticum [Made from common table salt] The Natrum muriaticum scans have a lot of flattened and smoothed out pieces, like they have been deflated [particularly look at the top middle piece in this scan- the piece that is circled]. One of the things the Natrum remedy treats is anemia, which can weaken the person and deflate the blood cells. The Natrum remedy also treats depression, which can cause a flat affect of a person's emotions; thus again, the scanned remedy chunks show the essence of the action of the remedy.

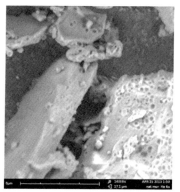

Natrum muriaticum 6x ©

Ruta graveolens [Made from the rue plant] - The Ruta graveolens remedy has scans that seem to have strong structures and smooth ridges. The Ruta remedy treats the bone coverings, tendons, ligaments and muscles. Strengthening these structures is a part of what the Ruta remedy does, thus, the remedy pieces show the essence of the remedy by looking strong. The Ruta remedy helps heal a bruised periosteum, the outer covering of the bone. Some of these bones have smooth ridges which are similar to the ridges in the Ruta scan structures. The scanned pictures show remedy formations that are strong and have an essence of strengthening. Plus, a lot of the pieces look similar to the bones, which shows the essence of structure of some of the bones. The Ruta remedy helps heal the periosteum, covering of bones. Below is an example of the radius bone of the arm which has the ridges that are comparable to the homeopathic Ruta remedy, which also has the ridges.

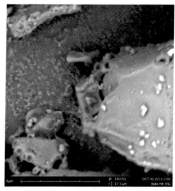

Ruta Graveolens 30c scan ©

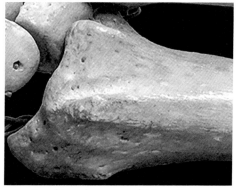

Radius bone of the Arm

Sepia [Made from the inky secretions of the cuttlefish] - The Sepia scans seem to show pock mark crevices in clusters, often on one side of the chunk. And there were also several flattened almost dish-shaped pieces. One of the target areas that the remedy works on is the hepatic portal system within the liver, which has round ducts, veins and arteries within it. These would look like pock mark crevices if seen from a slice of the liver. The mental/emotional aspects of the remedy are that the person can be irritable and 'touchy' with small outbursts of anxiety. This person would then become weak and have an indifferent, 'flattened' attitude. The scanned remedy shows a flattened side of the pieces, which shows the essence of the action of the remedy plus it looks similar to the target area, the liver slice which is where Sepia would perform some of its treatment.

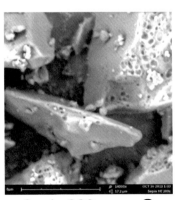

Sepia 200c scan©

Sulfur or Sulphur [Made from the mineral Sulphur] – Most of the Sulfur scanned pieces were very large in the size of their structures. Also, the structures of Sulfur scans have a variety of sizes, shapes and surfaces. This variety does seem to follow the Sulfur remedy's multiple actions. This is because it treats a variety of different problems. Sulfur is considered one of Dr. Hahnemann's most important remedies because it treats so many different problems. Thus, Sulfur is thought of as the largest remedy in its importance. The scans seem to show: the essence of the feelings; the large importance of the remedy; plus, the essence of the variety of its uses. It does this by the variety of shapes of the pieces, and the largeness of a lot of those pieces. The whole Sulfur pieces do not even fit in the scan and the smaller piece measures 11.1 micrometers, which is very large for 14,000x magnification.

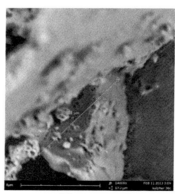

Sulfur 30c ©

Conclusion of the Addendum

It is my opinion that the ten remedies that were observed in this study, show in differing ways the essence, or footprint, of what is considered their vital force, the Chi, or the energy of their remedies. If more remedies are studied by other people, their essence probably will show the aspect of these remedies in the structures of the pieces that would show up in their scans.

Made in the USA
Lexington, KY
11 March 2018